Improving Vitality

PROVEN STRATEGIES TO DRAMATICALLY IMPROVE YOUR LIFESPAN WITH THE POWER OF NUTRITIONAL SUPPLEMENT AND RECIPES

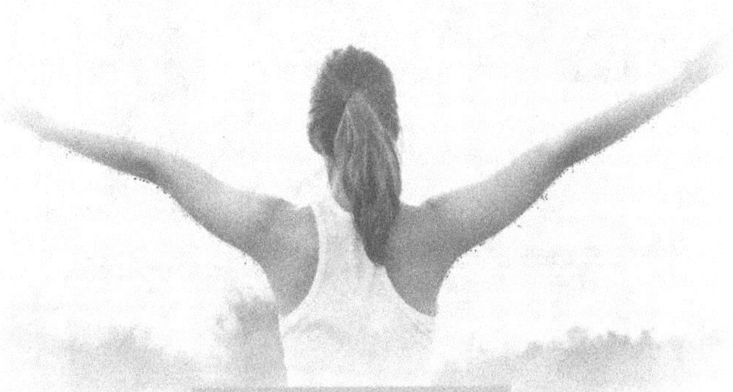

Catalina R. Lewis

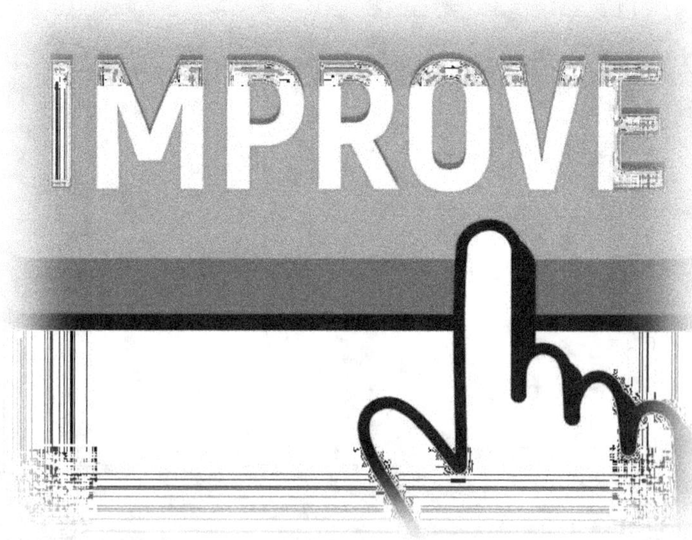
IMPROVE

TABLE OF CONTENT

Introduction 5

Supplements with Vitamins 7

Chapter 1: Vitamins and Your Health 10

Supplements and Your Well-Being 11

Chapter 2: Taking Supplements 14

A Lack of Vitamins 16

Getting Energy From Vitamins 18

Chapter 3: Getting The Right Amount of Vitamins ...20

Your System and Dietary Antioxidants 21

Chapter 4: Liquid Vitamin Supplements 24

Supplements with Antioxidants 26

Chapter 5: Supplements For Building Muscle 28

Supplements containing calcium 30

Chapter 6: What Are Vitamin Supplements? 32

Forms Of Vitamin Supplements 33

Different Supplements for Different Needs 34

Chapter 7: Common Contents Of Vitamin Supplements 36

Natural Vs. Synthetic Vitamin Supplements 37

Supplemental Vitamins' Advantages 38

Chapter 8: Good Food Health Vitamin Intake 40

Best Sources of Vitamins 41

Supplements of Mineral Vitamins 44

Recipes To Improve Vitality 46

Green smoothie..46

Avocado toast 46

Kale salad 47

Greek yogurt parfait 47

Quinoa bowl 48

Oatmeal...48

Overnight oats..49

Tofu scramble...49

Zucchini noodles...50

Veggie wraps...51

Conclusion...52

Take Only as Directed 52

Seek Your Doctor's Advice 52

Verify That It's Real...53

Introduction

People have been discussing and using nutritional supplements for a long time.

From their humble beginnings as natural herbs, these products have developed into a daily fad.

Supplements are more advanced than ever these days, and they come in a variety of formats, including liquid, pills, capsules, and teas. Though they aren't as well-liked as ones that are supplied professionally, some are nevertheless grown at home.

Generally speaking, people take nutritional supplements to supplement diets that are deficient in important minerals and nutrients. As mentioned above, they are available in a variety of forms and offer one or more essential components including vitamins, minerals, herbs, and amino acids. Nutritious supplements can be taken to improve your diet, but they aren't meant to take the place of meals.

There are numerous justifications for using dietary supplements. The surroundings are one of the causes. There are more toxins in the air, the water we consume, and the ecosystem as a whole due to the fast-changing meals that we consume. It is wise to take supplements and assist our systems in getting rid of the dangerous toxins because doing so requires our bodies to work twice as hard to eradicate these poisons.

Your body is also affected by stress. Stress can increase your body's vulnerability to a variety of conditions, including weakened immune systems.

As a result, taking supplements can help your body perform much better and rebuild your immune system. You can take a variety of nutritional supplements, such glyconutrients, to help you deal with stress.

The main cause of bad eating habits is the need for nutritional supplements. Those with hectic schedules occasionally overindulge in unhealthy food. Taking the time to eat a healthy meal might be extremely difficult at times.

When a nutritious meal is unavailable, we can always turn to supplements. They will improve our diets and provide us with the nutrients our bodies require for a variety of needs, including energy and wellness.

Those of us who work out or are athletic will require more nutrition for their bodies. Your body will require extra nutrients while you exercise or participate in sports. Supplements with protein, vitamins, and minerals are a few excellent examples. They can be found in a wide variety of foods, as well as in vitamins and dietary supplements.

Nutritious vitamins could be helpful if you're trying to reduce weight. When you go on a diet, you usually eat less and sometimes lose out on foods that are high in vital vitamins and minerals.

Conversely, your body won't be deficient in any vital vitamins or minerals if you take some dietary supplements. To make matters even better, you may get supplements that will support your weight loss efforts in addition to providing your body with all the nutrients it needs to do daily tasks.

Regardless of perspective, dietary supplements are excellent for a variety of purposes. You can get them online or at your neighborhood GNC or nutrition store. You can choose from a wide variety of supplements, providing all the necessary vitamins and nutrients.

Look no farther than nutritional supplements if you've been searching for a means to provide your body the vitamins, minerals, and nutrients it requires. They are reasonably priced, and you can choose from a wide range of cutting-edge products from numerous top manufacturers.

Supplements with Vitamins

Getting the right quantity of vitamins and nutrients from whole foods is crucial, but it may be somewhat challenging. In cases where a person's diet is inadequate in certain minerals, they resort to taking vitamins and supplements.

Given the popularity of vitamin supplements, there are numerous brands to pick from. There are thousands of supplements available every year, and consumers pay enormous sums of money to obtain the vitamins and supplements they require.

There are currently three main supplement administration methods available: liquid, capsules, and tablets. You should always choose one that dissolves easily and doesn't just pass through your system, even though each one is good on its own. Your vitamin will end up in the toilet and you will have wasted your money if it goes through your body.

Though there aren't many vitamins or supplements available in liquid form, liquid is thought to be the best. Some people prefer liquid, while others believe they taste like cough syrup. Liquid would be a fantastic substitute for tablets or capsules if you have trouble swallowing them.

Tablets are the most popular kind of supplement. Organic cement is used to manufacture tablets, which are subsequently shaped, Dissolving is the only downside in this case. Organic cements are necessary for tablets to dissolve correctly, but because they are more expensive, manufacturers often neglect to include them.

Supplement tablets with a coated shell are also available, albeit these are often found in the less expensive vitamin and supplement stores.

Many people prefer the capsule form of vitamin pills because they dissolve faster than other administration methods. You usually need to take two of them to acquire the same amount as comes with one tablet because they are not compacted like tablets are.

It is important to make sure you are getting the maximum levels of vitamins when using supplements. For people who are unable to eat the correct foods, vitamins are an excellent substitute for the minerals and nutrients contained in food.

Because vitamin supplements will give your body the amounts it needs for strenuous activity, they are also excellent for athletes and anyone looking for increased energy.

Vitamin supplements can be purchased online or from a nearby health food store like GNC. Among the most well-liked local retailers is GNC since they have an extensive selection of vitamins and supplements. Everything is available, including bodybuilding supplements and health vitamins.

They offer a wide range of manufacturers at deeply discounted prices, including well-known brands. GNC is a well-known brand in the vitamin and supplement industry, with over 100 locations across the US and millions of dollars in annual revenue.

See your doctor if you need to take vitamins or supplements but are unsure about which ones to take. Although vitamins and supplements are excellent sources of minerals and nutrients for your body, they should never take the place of diet in any way. You may be taking vitamins, but you still need to eat a balanced diet.

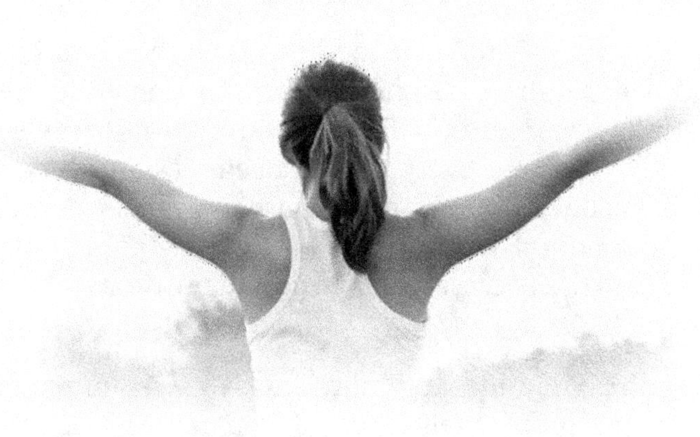

The benefits of taking vitamins and supplements will double if you can also maintain a healthy diet. You should always select your supplements carefully, ensuring sure you receive exactly what you require. Supplements and vitamins can be a great addition to a balanced diet if you choose them carefully.

Chapter 1: Vitamins and Your Health

As everyone knows these days, taking vitamins is a simple first step in living a healthy, disease-free life.

Vitamins were employed in conjunction with diets in the past, but they weren't quite as advanced as they are now. These days' vitamins are significantly more advanced and tailored to certain areas of your body and wellness.

Food does not provide your body with all the vitamins and nutrients it requires, despite the fact that some individuals may not be aware of this. Even if you eat a nutritious diet, your body won't get everything it needs to do its everyday tasks. If you'd want, you can purchase fine meals, but it's not the ideal solution in this kind of circumstance. You will never obtain the necessary vitamins and nutrients from your diet.

Getting the vitamins and nutrients you require may be considerably more challenging if you follow any kind of dietary restrictions. Those with food sensitivities in particular struggle even more to locate the quantity of vitamins. Being a picky eater might put you at a significant disadvantage when it comes to meeting your body's nutritional demands. Smaller appetites find it more difficult to eat the foods you need on a daily basis since they get full much faster.

Regardless of your perspective, food cannot provide your body with all it requires. You'll need to take vitamins and supplements in order to obtain the necessary vitamins, minerals, and nutrients. The simplest way to provide your body with what it needs is through vitamin supplements.

You can incorporate vitamins and supplements into your regular diet, but you'll need to choose them based on your needs and the components of your diet. While there are numerous vitamins that might aid you, B12 is one of the most crucial ones because it can boost your immune system and give you more energy. You should incorporate vitamins A, C, D, and E in your regular diet, among others.

Because they support numerous bodily processes, these vitamins are crucial. Among the most vital vitamins are C and E, which support healthy skin, healthy hair, and proper bodily function. You should make sure that your food includes the appropriate number of vitamins in order to maintain your body's optimal functioning. There are hundreds of vitamin supplements available online and in your area.

Selenium and colostrum are two other vitamins that you ought to incorporate into your daily diet because they are beneficial to your health. Your health and vitality will consistently stay at the peak of their abilities if you combine the appropriate vitamins with your diet.

Supplements and Your Well-Being

These days, a lot of people are attempting to improve their health. Everywhere you look, from newspapers to TV, you'll find articles about people and how ill they truly are. Even so, there

There are many different businesses that sell vitamins and supplements and promise to improve your health; you should do your homework to be sure you aren't wasting your money.

You should try a variety of vitamin supplements to determine which ones are ideal for you if you want to get healthier. Instead of only attempting a handful to see what works, you should consider all of the options. Since dieting can enhance your health the most, it's the best place to start. Dieting has the power to transform your body and improve your mood.

Many individuals these days consume far too much sugar and sweets, preferring refined goods to wholesome foods. While enjoying chocolate and sweets isn't always a terrible thing, you should never turn it into a habit. You can still indulge in your favorite foods, but you should consider the bigger picture and the health advantages of food as well.

You'll be eating healthily if you incorporate things like fruits, vegetables, and salads into your diet. Because it encourages muscle growth, protein is also good for your health. If you're serious about eating well but don't know where to begin, you should speak with a nutritionist. They will be able to advise you on how to begin and how to adopt a nutritious diet that will transform your life.

You'll probably find yourself wondering about vitamins and supplements and how much of an impact they make on your diet, even if you're attempting to eat healthily. Dieticians are the best people to ask these kinds of queries because they can respond to any inquiries you may have about vitamins.

Also, they may advise you on which supplements are best for your health and which ones you should eat. Since every person is unique, so are their demands and expectations, it is imperative to get professional counsel. In the event that you receive the guidance from a specialist, you'll be aware of the additions you can make to your diet. Should you attempt to handle everything on your own without seeking professional guidance, you may find yourself deficient in nutrients or using unnecessary medications.

Exercise has a significant impact on your nutrition and overall health. Exercise is the most beneficial thing you can do for your health, even though vitamins and supplements will help. You'll discover that you have more energy and feel better than you have in a long time if you exercise frequently and combine your diet with the correct supplements and vitamins.

Your doctor should always be consulted before beginning a new diet or hurriedly purchasing vitamin supplements to find out if he has any recommendations. you want to let him know what kind of exercise you intend to undertake and inquire about any potential health issues.

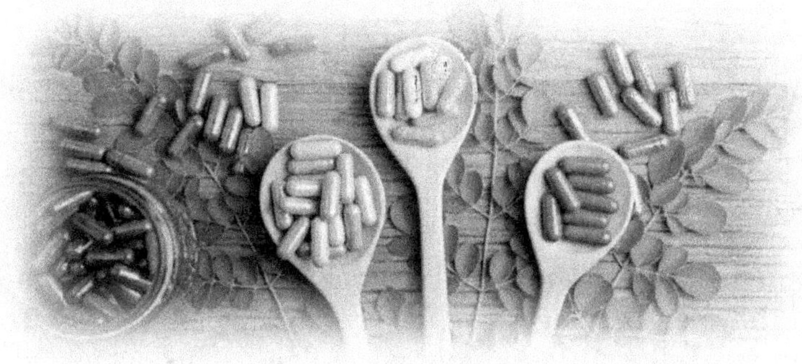

Adopting a healthy lifestyle is always beneficial, but you should always speak with your physician. You'll be able to start and approach getting into the best form of your life in this way.

Many people worldwide suffer from digestive system issues that make it difficult for them to absorb nutrients and digest their food.

This is a prevalent issue that is typically brought on by low stomach acid, toxins in the digestive tract, or insufficient development of the enzymes needed to aid in breakdown. While the aforementioned are the most frequent causes, there are more as well.

You can significantly improve digestive tract issues by gradually increasing your nutrient intake. The best method to enhance your digestion is to eat a diet high in organic matter, but you may also need to take supplements.

The fact that supplements don't require a prescription is their biggest feature. You can buy them online or at your neighborhood nutrition store after deciding which ones you want.

Supplements should ideally be taken with meals. Your body will be more able to absorb the nutrients at this time because the food will be stimulating to your digestive system. When utilizing time-released

supplements, you should take them with food to guarantee that they pass through your body smoothly and release the optimum quantity of vitamins and nutrients when your body needs them.

Water soluble vitamins are the easiest to use because they dissolve fast in the body and should be taken three times a day.

Fat-soluble vitamins are best absorbed when consumed alongside fat-containing foods. As the minerals and nutrients in food will complement vitamin supplements, you should always take your vitamins with meals.

Make sure any supplement you take is safe to use with other vitamin supplements as certain supplements have the potential to interfere with other supplements when they absorb.

The most popular vitamins are listed below, along with instructions on how to take them:

Vitamins A, D, and E: Foods high in fat or oil should always be consumed with these vitamins.

Vitamin B: To receive the most benefit, take vitamin B tablets as soon as you wake up. Additionally, you can take them with a full grain meal during the day.

Vitamin C: Never take vitamin C supplements on an empty stomach; instead, take them with meals.

Iron: Since iron is easily absorbed when taken with food, iron supplements should always be taken that way.

Multivitamins: Although you should always eat a modest meal along with the supplement, you can take multivitamins at any time.

You should make sure that you are obtaining the right vitamins and supplements in addition to maintaining a balanced diet.

Supplements can assist your body in getting the vitamins and minerals it requires, particularly on those days when you are unable to eat adequate food. Supplements can be really helpful when things get stressful in life.

Your body will be considerably healthier if you take vitamins as directed by your doctor and incorporate them into your diet. You can take a wide variety of vitamins and supplements, though which ones you take will depend on your goals.

Before making a purchase, you should always do your homework on a vitamin you're thinking about taking to make sure it will work for you.

A Lack of Vitamins

It is common knowledge that the human body need specific amounts of vitamins and minerals daily in order to maintain optimum function and health.

Your body can receive the vitamins it needs from a well-balanced diet, but if your diet is deficient in certain vitamins, issues and illnesses may develop. The advanced stage of vitamin insufficiency is typically when the symptoms of the condition become apparent.

For example, people who don't get enough of vitamins A, B1, or B2 may always feel exhausted and have decreased appetite. Chapped lips, other uncomfortable or painful habits, and mental and emotional strain are additional signs.

The most frequent causes of deficiency include inadequate nutrition, drunkenness, stress, and medications that prevent you from ingesting enough vitamins. You most likely don't get enough of the vitamins your body requires on a regular basis if you are always exhausted or lack energy.

Your doctor will probably offer vitamins and supplements to help you get what you need if you visit him and explain the situation. Never try to do too much at once or try to make up for lost time; you'll end up hurting yourself more than helping.

You may be eating a healthy diet, but you will still need to take supplements and vitamins. You should still use the appropriate vitamins and supplements to give your body the nourishment it needs, regardless of how healthily you eat.

In the event that your diet fails you, vitamins are an excellent backup supply because they will give your body the minerals and nutrients it needs.

You should take vitamins or supplements either before or after each meal. Make sure you always take the necessary amount of vitamins if you are deficient in any particular vitamin or vitamins, but lacking in a certain vitamin can negatively impact both your physical and overall well-being.

It's important to constantly search for supplements that include folic acid, vitamins B6, B12, D, and E. These well-known vitamins are also thought of as dietary supplements that can prevent cancer and maintain heart health. These vitamins work together to keep your body healthy, strengthen your immune system, and give you a renewed sense of well-being.

You will need to make an investment in vitamins and supplements if you want to stay healthy and maintain your body functioning properly. They are available online and at many local nutrition stores, many of which are very inexpensive.

It is important that you make sure you are taking and eating the correct foods, regardless of your age. Remember that vitamins are not meant to take the place of food; rather, they are meant to supplement your diet with extra nutrients and minerals.

You should always use vitamin supplements to provide your body with the nutrients it needs when you are unable to eat the correct foods. Vitamins and supplements are among the best purchases you can make, as Everybody's requires vitamins. When you consider it, the expenses are well worth it, even though they could mount up over time.

You can prevent a vitamin shortage and maintain your body's health for the price of vitamins and supplements. Vitamin deficiencies are quite frequent these days, but they don't have to be.

Getting Energy From Vitamins

The most common complaint patients have to doctors is that they are always tired or lack energy. It really isn't surprising that individuals are curious about the best vitamins and supplements they may take for energy, given these kinds of complaints. All vitamins are beneficial for maintaining your overall health and optimal physical function.

Folic acid is one of the most popular vitamins and supplements for energy. One B vitamin that has been shown to boost energy levels is folic acid. You can search for vitamins that give you energy, but it would be wiser to look for vitamins that also work effectively to combat exhaustion.

Supplements, vitamins, and minerals are excellent for preventing weariness and promoting alertness. Although many people are unaware of it, the vitamin known as NADH is quite effective for energy production. Those who regularly take vitamins would be quite pleased with the enhancement that NADH offers.

Despite the fact that its mechanism of action can be quite convoluted, it is frequently used to treat chronic fatigue.

Other vitamins that are excellent for supplying energy are gingko biloba and the MSM supplement.

Ginkgo biloba is a blood thinner, so if you use aspirin or another blood thinner, you should always talk to a physician or other qualified professional before using it. Despite the fact that it is regarded as an energy vitamin that can somewhat thin your blood when taken with aspirin. Blood thinners can cause lifelong health issues that can keep you from engaging in the activities you enjoy.

You should always get your doctor's advice before taking any vitamins for energy. You might not be able to take the vitamin of your choice if you have a major medical condition, such as a heart issue of any kind. This is the reason you should always seek the advice of your physician. Your doctor will be able to advise you on the kind of vitamins you should or shouldn't take after a few examinations and tests.

There are a lot of different energy sources available in the world of vitamins and supplements. There are many different vitamins available that can provide you with what you need, whether you're an athlete searching for extra energy or a senior citizen wishing to engage in more activities.

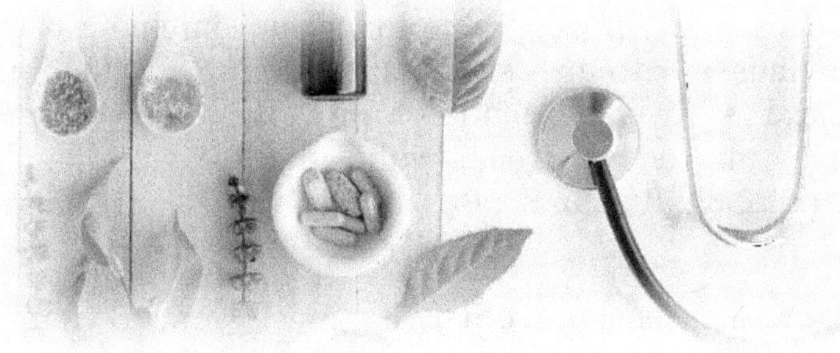

However, you should always speak with your doctor to find out if there are any vitamins you shouldn't be taking before you head out and explore your alternatives.

Chapter 3: Getting The Right Amount of Vitamins

Every day, if you eat well-balanced meals, your body will receive all the vitamins and minerals it needs to function.

We all require vitamins to stay healthy and avoid disease, even though our dietary demands are diverse. Since vitamins have been around for hundreds of years, they have given us the means to lead healthy lives.

Despite the wide variety of vitamins available, your body requires a specific quantity of each to remain healthy. Vitamins are categorized into numerous categories, such as A, B, C, and E. Each of these vitamins has a specific function that benefits your body and your overall health, making them all very vital.

Vitamin B are the most varied group of vitamins in terms of kind. This vitamin, which was found by combining many compounds, is extremely significant. Because the vitamin B complex is so diverse, scientists have separated the vitamin into eight distinct subgroups within the B vitamin family. The B1, B2, B3, B5, B6, B7, B9, and B12 varieties are among them.

Similar to deficiencies in other vitamin classes, a B vitamin shortage can lead to a variety of ailments, including anemia, diarrhea, weight loss, weakness, stress, and dementia. Given that the entire family contributes to your body, having a B vitamin shortage is bad for everybody. You should always take action as soon as possible if you are deficient in any of the variations of this vitamin.

The B vitamin family as a whole will help you have faster metabolism, healthier skin, and an enhanced immune system. They can also assist you in retaliating against stress and depression, which is something that we could all benefit from.

Regardless of perspective, this vitamin family has the potential to significantly enhance life as we know it. The B family of vitamins is among the most vital, even though other vitamins are also necessary for a healthy diet. Because they significantly enhance your body and your health, all of these vitamins ought to be a part of your regular diet.

You might not be getting enough of the B vitamin family, even if you eat a healthy diet. Should this be the situation, you ought to research vitamin supplements that provide you with the necessary amounts of B vitamins. Lack of B vitamins can have detrimental effects on your body and health, even if you may not be aware of this.

You will know that you are getting what you require for a healthy existence if you choose wisely and obtain some B vitamin supplements.

Your System and Dietary Antioxidants

Many of the meals high in antioxidants that we eat come from plants, despite the fact that many people are unaware of this. Broccoli, cauliflower, tomatoes, and peppers are a few examples of vegetables that are fantastic choices and have many health benefits. Because they are higher in what are known as phytonutrients, colorful vegetables are the ones you should always choose to eat.

The compound's called phytonutrients are present in the skins of a variety of fruits and vegetables and are responsible for the color, flavor, and aroma of the meal. The greatest kinds of antioxidant foods that you may discover anyplace are, quite simply, phytonutrients. The high amount of antioxidant value that coq10 gives is ideal if you're searching for a supplement. The issue with fruits and vegetables, while being the best sources of antioxidants, is that they are grown using chemical pesticides, herbicides, and fertilizers.

Studies conducted over the years have demonstrated that fruits and vegetables cultivated organically have a higher content of antioxidants than produce that has been produced commercially. It can be difficult to eat healthily in today's hectic environment, and we can't always consume organic fruits and veggies. If you are unable to obtain organic fruits or other foods high in antioxidants, you might consider taking nutritional supplements that provide you with the necessary phytonutrients in your diet.

Phytonutrient-containing supplements do offer an edge over some vegetables, including carrots, which can cause dangerously high blood sugar levels. The phytonutrients present in supplements are derived from pigments that have been extracted to concentrate nutrients. This means that the nutrients found in antioxidant foods are maximized, while calories and sugar are excluded.

It's important to remember that fruits and vegetables are healthy foods. They are rich in antioxidants, although commercially made varieties typically contain unhealthful chemicals and other substances. Antioxidant supplements lack the high sugar and calorie content of canned fruits and vegetables. You may get the levels you require from the supplements without any added chemicals, sweets, or calories. You won't have to worry about consuming anything unhealthy in this method.

Antioxidant-rich foods are the foundation of a healthy diet for your body, no matter how you slice it. Antioxidants are present in a variety of diets, with fruits and vegetables having the highest concentrations.

Meat and steak provide a wealth of other health advantages, like protein, and are also excellent providers of antioxidants. If you're unable to consume foods high in antioxidants, you can always rely on supplements to provide you with the necessary amount to maintain your health.

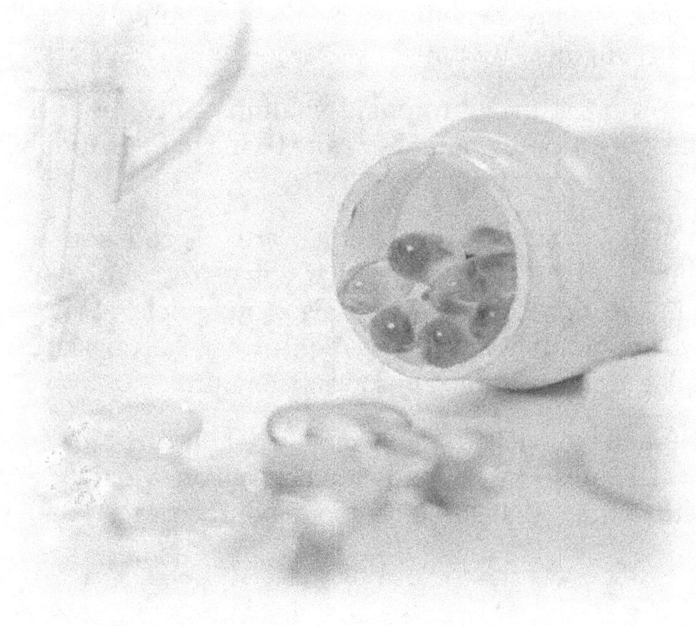

Chapter 4: Liquid Vitamin Supplements

Liquid vitamin pills were unheard of several years ago.

The best way to take supplements used to be with tablets and pills. Even though they were highly regarded, some people would just pass them through their bodies without experiencing any benefits since they couldn't enter the bloodstream quickly enough.

Manufacturers turned to liquid vitamins since the market was begging for more and they were trying to figure out how to improve the vitamin.

Even while fruits and vegetables are a good source of vitamins and nutrients, they are not nearly sufficient to sustain life on their own. It's also impossible to eat the proper amount that our bodies require on a daily basis, even though they contain the appropriate amount.

The human stomach is simply unable to hold all of the fruits and vegetables that an individual need on a daily basis, despite the fact that some people may prefer to eat a lot of them.

You'll need to take vitamin supplements in order to receive the proper amount of minerals and nutrients. For a very long time, taking supplements has been the best approach to give your body the minerals and nutrition it needs.

Vitamins in pills and tablets can provide you with what you need, but they don't get the essential nutrients into your body quickly enough. Vitamin supplements in liquid form quickly enter your bloodstream and body, showing results in a shorter amount of time.

You can also live a better life and enhance your health by using liquid vitamin supplements. You will never be able to eat a nutritious meal all the time, no matter how strict your diet is.

It can be challenging to receive the nutrition you need due to busy lifestyles, which is where supplements really shine. No matter where you are or how busy your day gets, you can always take liquid supplements.

The fact that liquid vitamin pills are all-inclusive is another fantastic feature. Your body will typically absorb 20% of the nutrients in pills and capsules that contain supplements. Conversely, liquid vitamin supplements are more readily absorbed by your body and reach your important parts more quickly.

Compared to pills or tablets, they are significantly easier to digest because they are liquid. As a result, liquid supplements are starting to replace pills and tablets.

You want to consider liquid supplements if you've been searching for the ideal vitamin supplements for your body. There are numerous manufacturers out there that can provide you with state-of-the-art vitamins for your body and well-being.

You can take them with meals in the same manner that you would pills and tablets. In this manner, you'll obtain the necessary amounts of protein and other nutrients from food, as well as the vital vitamins and other nutrients your body need from liquid vitamin supplements.

Supplements with Antioxidants

Antioxidants are essential for maintaining a healthy lifestyle and making lifestyle improvements. There are several natural antioxidant supplements available that won't harm you and can support a healthy lifestyle. Although taking supplements is the best way to ensure that you are getting the recommended quantities of antioxidants, you may also eat a variety of foods that are high in antioxidants.

One of the advantages of increasing your intake of antioxidants through diet and supplements is that it will protect your cells. By shielding your cells from harm, antioxidants can help prevent disease.

Your body may frequently be deficient in vitamins, which will slow down your recovery from illnesses or injuries. You will be able to detect the differences if your body contains the appropriate amounts of vitamins and antioxidants.

Antioxidant supplements are generally available as herbal or natural products, and they will be very beneficial to your body. They also offer many other advantages, like lowering blood clotting, avoiding numerous illnesses, and increasing libido. Good nutrition and diet management are vital aspects of life; therefore, you should always take care of your health and make sure you eat healthily.

There are supplements available that aren't synthetic and are perfect for maintaining your health. Unlike manufactured vitamins, your body can readily absorb them. It's common knowledge that synthetic supplements penetrate slowly, meaning it may take a while to notice any kind of benefit.

Conversely, non-synthetic ingredients provide nearly instant benefits because they are readily absorbed by the body and have no negative side effects.

Remember that maintaining a nutritious diet is still necessary, even if you are taking vitamins that include antioxidants. Even though the supplements will provide you with more vitamins, you still need to eat food that has the necessary minerals and vitamins.

If you are unable to eat the correct foods that contain these valuable nutrients, you can also utilize antioxidant-containing vitamins and supplements.

You should constantly make sure that antioxidant-containing foods and supplements are a part of your diet, for many reasons. You run the danger of illness or other negative consequences if you don't consume enough antioxidants.

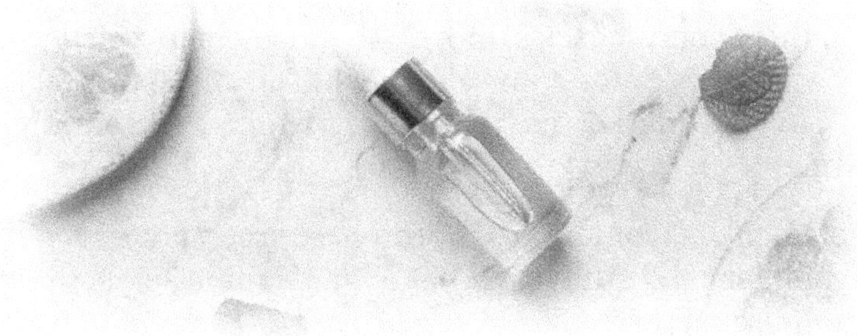

Because of the many health benefits that antioxidants provide, you should make sure you are getting enough of them in your diet. All you have to do is make sure you are eating healthily and making every effort to lead a healthy lifestyle. There are many different vitamins and supplements available that include them.

Chapter 5: Supplements For Building Muscle

If you were to stroll into your neighborhood health and nutrition store in search of muscle-building supplements, you most likely would be taken aback by the sheer number of options available to you.

Selecting the right supplements to support your goals can be a bit difficult with so many options available. There are several supplements available to aid with muscle growth, but some might not be the best for your objectives.

The first thing to remember is that, while they can speed up the process, muscle building supplements are not always necessary to gain muscle.

As long as you exercise, these supplements can help you strengthen your muscles more. They can help you build muscle and help your muscles heal. The most well-liked items on the market include multivitamins, protein, and creatine.

Supplements containing protein are favored by bodybuilders and athletes. It has a lot of amino acids, which aid in muscular growth.

Whichever diet, supplement, or plan you choose, you should always go for one that is high in protein. Two grams of protein for every pound of body weight is the recommended intake. Protein is available as pills, powder, or even bars.

Also, you should confirm that the protein supplement you choose contains eggs, whey, and soy. The best supplement is whey protein because it has all the ingredients you need to begin gaining muscle.

Another useful supplement is creatine, which can help you gain muscular growth and speed up your muscles' recuperation. creatine increases muscle pumps, which enables you to perform more repetitions with greater weight.

It is typically necessary for you to undergo a loading phase of one week for creatine. After loading it, you should utilize it in cycles, utilizing it for a few weeks and then taking a few weeks off. You should always adhere to the directions on the label provided by the manufacturer if you want to get the most out of creatine.

Another fantastic supplement is micro-vitamins, which are especially beneficial for people whose regular diets don't provide them with enough minerals and vitamins. Getting a healthy dinner might be rather difficult, even with the best of intentions, if you have a busy or demanding schedule.

You may provide your body with the vitamins and minerals it needs by include vitamin supplements in your diet. When trying to gain muscle, it's important to always take the right supplements and, in the event that you can't have a good meal, use protein bars and smoothies.

All of us would like to gain more muscle. You should have the required supplements in addition to putting in a lot of effort and exercise on your part.

It won't take long for you to see the muscular growth if you use the appropriate supplements. Supplements will expedite the process of muscular growth.

There are numerous manufacturers and brands available. These supplements are available online and locally, providing you with a plethora of fantastic offers to choose from.

You should take muscle building pills if you work out and want to gain more muscle mass in your body. They taste fantastic, they function very well, and they will help you achieve your goals of being healthy and gaining muscle.

Supplements containing calcium

You will find that calcium is crucial for the rest of your life. Getting the recommended quantities of calcium is crucial during some of the most significant periods of your life, including childhood, breastfeeding, and pregnancy. Calcium helps kids' teeth and bones grow and keeps blood clots from forming. In adulthood, calcium aids in the prevention of osteoporosis.

If you are considering taking calcium supplements or already do, you should take them with a large glass of liquid—ideally water—either before or after your meal. Make careful to fully chew the pills before swallowing them if you're using chewable calcium supplements.

If you find it difficult to chew, you should always dissolve them in a glass of juice or water and then take a steady sip. Remember that taking other medications right after taking calcium supplements can cause problems because they can conflict with other prescriptions you may be taking.

Even though calcium supplements are great for supporting healthy bone and tooth development, you should always confirm that you can take them before buying. Before using calcium supplements, those with lung disease, kidney stones, stomach issues, or diarrhea should always see a doctor to make sure they won't worsen their condition.

It is advisable to inform your doctor if you are pregnant if you use calcium supplements or are considering doing so because these supplements have the potential to enter breast milk.

In general, anyone can take calcium supplements; nevertheless, excessive dosages may result in unusual and unfavorable side effects. A dry mouth, nausea, vomiting, constipation, and appetite loss are possible side effects of taking heavy amounts of calcium supplements. You should get in touch with your doctor right away if you begin to experience any of the issues listed above.

Tell your doctor about any additional medications you are taking as well as any family medical history of illnesses when you call.

Supplements containing calcium can be taken by anybody, but in rare circumstances, they can have negative effects. Although they are extremely uncommon, side effects might occur and may discourage some people from using these supplements.

Calcium supplements are essential if you've been experiencing issues with your bones or if you just want to maintain the health of your bones. They are available online and in nearby health food stores like GNC.

They won't break the bank, and you'll have the assurance that your bones will continue to be strong and healthy. You can also incorporate them into your regular diet, but you should first consult your doctor to make sure they won't pose any risks.

Chapter 6: What Are Vitamin Supplements?

For the body to function correctly and to remain healthy, among other reasons, vitamins are necessary for everyone.

The most frequent sources of vitamins that our bodies absorb are the meals we eat.

Every meal has a specific vitamin, and the quantity of a vitamin we consume is determined by how much of that item we eat. However, the majority of the time, the vitamins they offer are insufficient. We therefore require vitamin supplements.

As the name implies, a vitamin supplement enriches a person's diet with the vitamins required for the body's regular functions.

Also, those who are lacking in a certain vitamin due to their current health (such as pregnant women) or the type of food they follow (vegetarians), require these supplements.

The most often occurring vitamins in supplements include, among others, vitamins A, B1, B2, B3, B6, and C. These vitamins can be purchased as pills, gels, or capsules, among other forms.

According to some, each form is more successful than the others at supplying the body with the necessary vitamins. by giving us the vital vitamins that we might not be getting from the foods we eat, vitamin supplements can help us live better, stronger lives. If we take one tablet a day, our bodies can benefit much from it.

Forms Of Vitamin Supplements

There are various vitamin supplement forms on the market, despite the tablet being the most widely used one. The majority of these alternative forms, if not all of them, assert that their vitamin delivery to the body is superior to that of other forms.

Let's examine each of them more closely to see how successful they actually are:

Tablet: As previously indicated, this is the most common form of vitamin supplementation. Additionally, a lot of people choose to get their vitamins in this manner due to its accessibility.

Some, on the other hand, dislike this choice since the body finds it difficult to absorb. As a result, a large portion of it is wasted along with the pee, which is sometimes mockingly called "expensive urine."

Capsule: The capsule and the tablet are extremely similar. The size of them is the only distinction between them, as tablets are significantly larger than capsules. Some choose to take their supplements in the form of capsules as a result.

Softgel: With a softer shell, this is quite similar to a tablet. Because the body absorbs it more readily than a pill, people prefer it.

Liquid: Of the three forms previously stated, this one is thought to be absorbed by the body the best. Liquids promise 90% absorption, but pills and capsules only absorb 40–50% of their contents.

Different Supplements for Different Needs

You will see a wide variety of vitamin supplements on the shelves of your neighborhood health and medicine store.

Here is some useful information to offer you an overview of the most popular vitamin supplements on the market in case you're wondering what each of them accomplishes.

Multivitamins

Perhaps the most popular vitamin supplement on the market is this one. The necessary vitamins and minerals are provided by one tablet from — you already know what comes next. A to Zinc.

Vitamin B Complex

contains many B vitamins (B1, B2, B3, B5, B6, B7, and B12) in combination, and it is occasionally supplemented with other vitamins. Its advantages include stress reduction and strong bones, hair, and skin.

Vitamin C

Known by another name, ascorbic acid, this is typically used to strengthen one's immune system. Furthermore, contrary to popular belief, this vitamin can lessen the symptoms of colds but not prevent them.

Vitamin E

People who wish to stop, reverse, or at least slow down the aging process are big fans of this vitamin. Beyond that, though, vitamin E offers a plethora of additional advantages, including strengthening the immune system, lowering the chance of prostate cancer, and relieving female menstruation cramps.

There you have it. the most widely available vitamin supplements available. We hope the knowledge is helpful to you and that you may put it to use the next time you shop at your preferred health and medicine store.

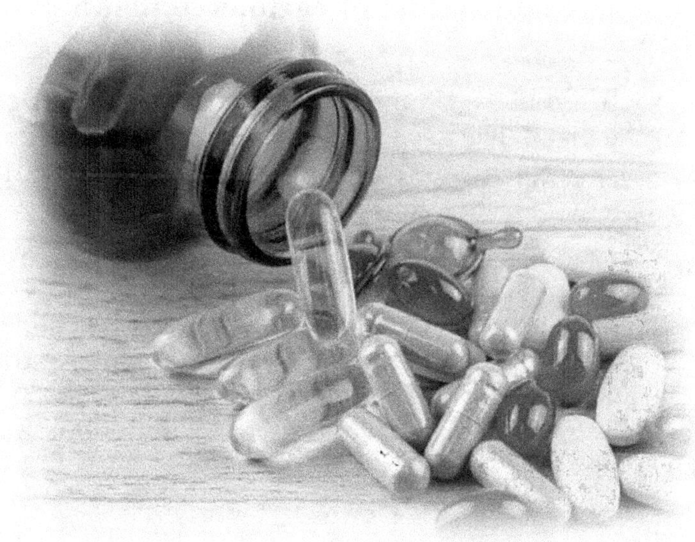

Chapter 7: Common Contents Of Vitamin Supplements

The vitamins included in each pill are known to anyone who takes vitamin supplements and has ever looked at the bottles or cartons containing the supplements.

What exactly do those vitamins do, though? Really, do you have to take them? The most popular vitamins that are often included in supplements are listed here, along with an explanation of their functions.

Vitamin A

This vitamin, which is frequently present in leafy vegetables as well as foods including eggs, liver, broccoli, papaya, carrots, and broccoli, helps maintain healthy eyes. A persistent loss of vision may result from a vitamin B12 shortage.

Vitamin B1

This vitamin is also known as thiamine. It maintains normal function of the heart, neurological system, and digestive tract. In addition, thiamine plays a role in the physical maturation and development of an individual. Among other things, beef, pork, almonds, and legumes are good providers of this vitamin.

Vitamin B2

This vitamin, often referred to as riboflavin, is crucial for the metabolism of proteins, lipids, and carbohydrates in addition to energy. Typical sources of this vitamin are green vegetables, cheese, and milk. Among other signs of a vitamin B12 shortage include sore throats, mouth ulcers, and cracked lips.

Vitamin C

This vitamin, which is sometimes referred to as ascorbic acid, is said to offer numerous advantages. Increasing immune function and reducing disease symptoms are a couple of them. It's a well-known antioxidant as well. Inadequate intake of this vitamin can result in scurvy, which can cause tooth loss and ultimately death.

Natural Vs. Synthetic Vitamin Supplements

Nowadays, a lot of individuals are obsessed with natural products. They claim that compared to those made in labs, they are safer and more effective.

In the realm of vitamin supplements, the same discussion is ongoing. There are those who support synthetic supplements and those who advocate for natural supplements.

But do the two actually differ from one another? Both yes and no. Why? The solutions are given below.

The primary distinction between the two is that one is made in a lab, while the other is extracted from a natural source.

There isn't a conclusive study that supports the claims made by proponents of natural products that theirs is superior since it is purer.

And there's the difference in pricing. The claim that so-called natural products cost more than their synthetic equivalents is no longer news.

There's no need for a dispute unless evidence proving one is more effective than the other is provided, even though the price difference can be explained by the methods they have prepared.

However, since people will always prefer one thing over another, the argument about which is superior may never end.

But the amount of vitamins that are actually present in these supplements matters more than the source or the method of production.

Certain natural supplements contain extra components that reduce their intended effect, whereas synthetic supplements are overly packed with vitamins, which decreases their efficacy.

Supplemental Vitamins' Advantages

It's common knowledge that eating a nutritious diet will keep us healthy and enable us to pursue our interests. But it's just not enough to sustain us at the highest level of performance every single day.

Vitamin supplements are necessary to provide us the extra push we need to complete our everyday chores and maintain optimal bodily functions.

Supplements containing vitamins give us the critical nutrients our bodies require. In addition, it makes up for any vitamins we might be missing from our diet, both when we eat and when we don't.

However, if we examine the vitamins contained in a standard supplement more closely, we can discover the unique advantages that each vitamin provides for our bodies. There is vitamin C, to start.

In a supplement, it often has the greatest dosage. This specific vitamin is well known for strengthening our immune systems, but it also helps lessen cold and other illness-related symptoms.

A sufficient amount of vitamin A from the supplement aids in maintaining eye health in the interim. It is crucial to include this vitamin in the supplement's formulation because any shortage can result in blindness.

a deeper examination of the vitamins included in supplements and an understanding of their advantages enable us to recognize their significance for our day-to-day existence.

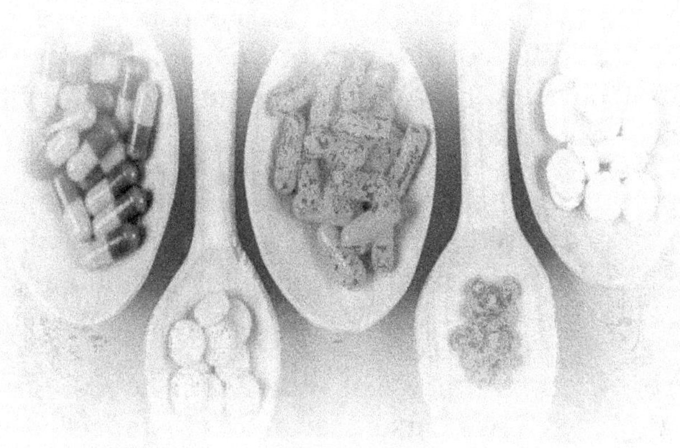

With the help of vitamin supplements, we can live healthier lives when combined with exercise and a balanced diet.

Chapter 8: Good Food Health Vitamin Intake

Understanding what makes for a healthy vitamin intake from food is crucial.

For most vitamins that are considered a desirable food health vitamin consumption, the Federal Drug Administration establishes a recommended daily allowance.

These numbers change according on an individual's age, gender, and other characteristics, thus a young woman's recommended daily intake of vitamins for optimal health will differ from a guy in his seventies.

The nutritional labeling of certain items includes the levels of vitamins that are necessary for good health. A person should take into consideration this labeling as it aids guarantee that they are getting the right amount of vitamins from their food intake for wellness.

In the pursuit of a healthy vitamin intake, nutritional data is frequently expressed as a percentage of the daily allowance of each vitamin and mineral. This helps evaluate the food's worth.

As part of their intake of nutritious foods, healthful vitamins, there are also certain substances that an individual may wish to limit in their diet. Once more, a person can determine how high a product contains these unwanted substances by looking at the nutritional label of particular items.

Even while salt and fat are not precisely vitamins, they are foods that one may wish to limit as part of their excellent dietary health vitamin intake.

When most people use the phrase "vitamin," they really mean "nutrients," and food makers know that when consumers think about their consumption of vitamins for optimum health, they also consider minerals and other elements.

Another component that is becoming more widely recognized is fiber, which is required for a healthy vitamin intake and forms a crucial part of a balanced diet.

A person needs to be even more mindful of their intake of healthy foods and vitamins if they are on a restricted diet for whatever reason.

Naturally, different meals contain different nutrients from one another. This also applies to vitamins, so if a person is unable to eat particular foods, it may be more difficult for them to get the recommended daily dose of vitamins for optimal health.

For those who cannot get enough vitamins from their regular diet, vitamin supplements can play a crucial role in a healthy vitamin consumption.

It's also important to keep in mind that a person's lifetime vitamin requirements for excellent meals depend on their overall health.

Best Sources of Vitamins

The question of which vitamin is the best is hotly contested. Every vitamin has a unique set of vital properties that support overall health and wellbeing.

It is not possible to declare one of these to be the best vitamin. Nonetheless, certain meals offer the highest concentrations of vitamins.

For each vitamin, there are different best sources. To make sure that you are getting the recommended levels of every vitamin, it is crucial to maintain a balanced diet.

To serve as a reference, it could be helpful to enumerate the best sources of each vitamin.

- The best sources of vitamin A include liver, eggs, butter, milk, and yellow and dark green fruits and vegetables.
- Brewer's yeast, whole grains, blackstrap molasses, brown rice, organ meats, and egg yolks are the best sources of vitamin B1.
- The best sources of vitamin B2 include organ meats, whole grains, legumes, nuts, brewer's yeast, and blackstrap molasses.
- The best sources of vitamin B3 include lean meats, chicken, fish, peanuts, milk, rice bran, and potatoes.
- Egg yolks, organ meats, brewer's yeast, wheat germ, soybeans, salmon, and legumes are the best sources of vitamin B4.
- The best sources of vitamin B5 include organ meats, egg yolks, whole grains, legumes, wheat germ, salmon, and brewer's yeast.
- The best sources of vitamin B6 include whole grains, meats, organ meats, brewer's yeast, blackstrap molasses, and wheat germ.
- Egg yolks, liver, unpolished rice, brewer's yeast, sardines, legumes, and whole grains are the best sources of vitamin B7.

- The best sources of vitamin B8 include brewer's yeast, meat, milk, nuts, vegetables, citrus fruits, whole grains, and molasses.
- The best sources of vitamin B9 include dark green leafy vegetables, milk, oysters, salmon, root vegetables, and organ meats.
- The best sources of vitamin B12 are seafood, poultry, eggs, cheese, milk, lamb, bananas, kelp, and peanuts.
- The best sources of vitamin B13 are liquid whey and root vegetables.
- The best sources of vitamin B15 include brown rice, brewer's yeast, rare steaks, sunflower, pumpkin, and sesame seeds.
- Whole kernels of apricots, apples, cherries, peaches, and plums are the best sources of vitamin B17.
- Citrus, cabbage family, chilli peppers, berries, melons, asparagus, and rose hips are the best sources of vitamin C.
- The best sources of vitamin D include organ meats, milk, egg yolks, sardines, herring, sprouting seeds, and sunflower seeds.
- The best sources of vitamin E include organ meats, cold-pressed oils, eggs, wheat germ, sweet potatoes, molasses, and almonds.
- Sunflower seeds, butter, and vegetable oils are the best sources of vitamin F.
- The best sources of vitamin K are egg yolks, safflower oil, cauliflower, blackstrap molasses, and green leafy vegetables.
- Legumes, soybeans, and pinto beans are the best sources of vitamin Q.

- The best sources of vitamin T include egg yolks, butter, sesame seeds, and raw seeds.
- Leafy vegetables, sauerkraut, and raw cabbage are the best sources of vitamin V.

Supplements of Mineral Vitamins

Most mineral vitamin supplements are manufactured with chemicals instead of natural ingredients. On the other hand, the market for natural mineral vitamin supplements is steadily expanding.

This is because there is a lot of disagreement over whether chemical mineral vitamins have a longer-term detrimental effect than a good one.

The truth is that regular food particles absorb nutrients more readily than artificial mineral supplements. The mineral vitamin sector is always trying to make goods that are easier for the body to process and hence more advantageous.

Occasionally, a new, "more bioavailable" version of a vitamin or mineral is developed by the industry. In order to get around this, a ton of mineral vitamins have been created, combining vitamins and minerals with other components to make them easier for the body to absorb. Iron is frequently mixed with other elements to create iron gluconate, which increases the mineral vitamin supplement's absorbability.

For the body to absorb the necessary amount of a nutrient from a mineral vitamin supplement, the amount must be significantly higher than it would be in a more natural form. This might clearly result in issues when the high dosages of the required mineral vitamin supplement are consuming a poisonous level of that specific nutrient. For this reason, it is crucial that a

A person should see a health practitioner rather to just ingesting large amounts of all the mineral and vitamin supplements that are promoted on television. It is also beneficial to be informed about the advancements occurring in the mineral vitamin supplement sector, since new and improved formulations are continuously being created.

Culturing the raw ingredients with yeast cells is one technique pioneered by mineral vitamin makers to help enhance absorption. When the yeast is fully digested, the body may absorb the necessary minerals from these "food state" mineral vitamins up to four times more easily.

Of course, a person's diet has an impact on their requirement for mineral and vitamin supplements. Without a question, wherever possible, it is far better for a person to get the nutrients they need from their food rather than by taking mineral or vitamin supplements.

While it is not advised to use many of the available supplements over the long term, there are times when someone may need to take mineral vitamin supplements temporarily.

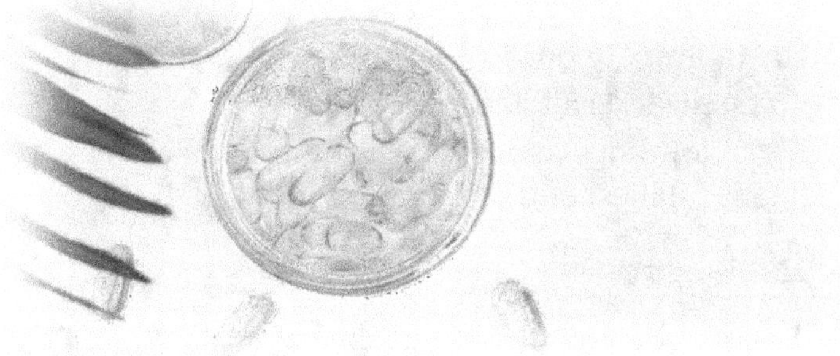

Recipes To Improve Vitality

Green smoothie

Ingredients

- One cup of spinach leaves
- Half a cucumber, cut into slices and peel
- half an avocado
- One banana
- One cup of green grapes
- One cup of coconut water
- Cubes of ice (optional)

Guidelines:

- Blend spinach, avocado, cucumber, banana, grapes, and coconut water.
- Blend till creamy and smooth.
- If desired, add ice cubes and mix one more.
- After pouring into a glass, savor your wholesome green smoothie!

Avocado toast

- 2 pairs of wholegrain slices
- One mature avocado
- To taste, add salt and pepper.
- Extra toppings at your discretion: Poached egg, red pepper flakes, and cherry tomatoes

Guidelines:

- As desired, toast the bread slices.

- Mash the ripe avocado in a basin with salt and pepper to taste while the bread is toasting.
- Over the toast, equally distribute the mashed avocado.
- Add the seasonings and toppings of your choice.
- Enjoy your delectable avocado toast after serving!

Kale salad

- four cups of finely chopped kale
- one cup of cherry tomatoes, halved
- Half a cup of crumbled feta cheese
- 1/4 cup finely sliced red onion
- 1/4 cup of dressing for a balsamic vinaigrette

Guidelines:

- Chopped kale, cherry tomatoes, feta cheese, and red onion should all be combined in a big bowl.
- Over the salad, drizzle the balsamic vinaigrette dressing.
- Mix the salad until it's evenly covered.
- Give it a few minutes to settle so the flavors can combine.
- Present and relish a revitalizing kale salad!

Greek yogurt parfait

- One cup of Greek yogurt
- Half a cup of granola
- ½ cup of mixed berries, including raspberries, blueberries, and strawberries

Directions

- Arrange Greek yogurt, granola, and mixed berries in a glass or bowl.
- Layers should be repeated until the container is full.
- For sweetness, drizzle some honey over the top.
- Enjoy this delicious Greek yogurt parfait right away by serving it immediately!

Quinoa bowl

- One cup of cooked quinoa
- Half a cup of rinsed and drained black beans
- half a cup of kernels of corn
- quartered cherry tomatoes, half a cup
- 1/4 cup chopped cilantro with lime wedges as a garnish

Guidelines:

- Cooked quinoa, black beans, corn, cherry tomatoes, and cilantro should all be combined in a bowl.
- Mixing the components well is necessary.
- For added taste, squeeze some lime wedges over the quinoa bowl.
- Present and savor a tasty and nourishing quinoa bowl!

Oatmeal

- One cup of rolled oats
- Two cups of milk (vegan or dairy)
- One spoonful of maple syrup
- Half a teaspoon of extract from vanilla
- Extra toppings at your discretion: banana slices, chopped almonds, and berries

<u>Guidelines:</u>

- Milk and rolled oats should be combined in a saucepan.
- Cook the oats over medium heat, stirring from time to time, until it reaches the consistency you like.
- Add vanilla extract and maple syrup, and stir.
- Take it off the fire and let it to cool a little.
- After adding your preferred toppings, savor a warm cup of oatmeal!

Overnight oats

- Half a cup of rolled oats
- Half a cup of milk (vegan or dairy)
- half a cup of Greek yogurt
- One spoonful of chia seeds
- One tablespoon of honey
- Extra toppings at your discretion: nuts and sliced fruits

<u>Guidelines:</u>

- Roll the oats, milk, Greek yogurt, chia seeds, and honey into a jar or other container.
- Be sure to thoroughly stir to incorporate all of the ingredients.
- Refrigerate overnight with a cover on.
- Stir well and top with your preferred toppings in the morning.
- Make overnight oats for a quick and wholesome breakfast!

Tofu scramble

- One block of crumbly firm tofu

- One tablespoon of olive oil
- One sliced bell pepper
- half an onion diced
- One cup of spinach leaves
- One tsp of turmeric
- To taste, add salt and pepper.

Guidelines:

- In a pan set over medium heat, warm the olive oil.
- Saute the bell pepper and sliced onion till they get tender.
- Add the tofu crumbles, turmeric, salt, and pepper to the pan.
- Stirring occasionally, cook the tofu until it takes on the texture of scrambled eggs.
- When the spinach begins to wilt, add it.
- Serve the hot tofu scramble and savor a plant-based morning choice!

Zucchini noodles

- Two big spiralized zucchini
- One tablespoon of olive oil
- two minced garlic cloves
- To taste, add salt and pepper.
- Add some optional parmesan cheese as a garnish.

Guidelines:

- In a pan set over medium heat, warm the olive oil.
- When aromatic, add the minced garlic and sauté it.
- When the zucchini noodles are heated through, add them to the pan and stir.
- Add pepper and salt for seasoning.

- If desired, sprinkle some Parmesan cheese on top.
- For a quick and healthful zucchini noodle dish, serve right away!

Veggie wraps

- Whole-grain tortillas
- Hummus
- cucumber slices
- bell peppers, sliced (many hues)
- Carrots, shredded
- slices of avocado
- crisp lettuce leaves

Guidelines:

- Arrange the whole-grain wrappers in a tidy manner.
- On each wrapper, spread a layer of hummus.
- Top each wrap with a slice of cucumber, bell peppers, shredded carrots, avocado, and lettuce.
- Tightly roll the wraps after folding the sides.
- If desired, cut in half and fasten with toothpicks.

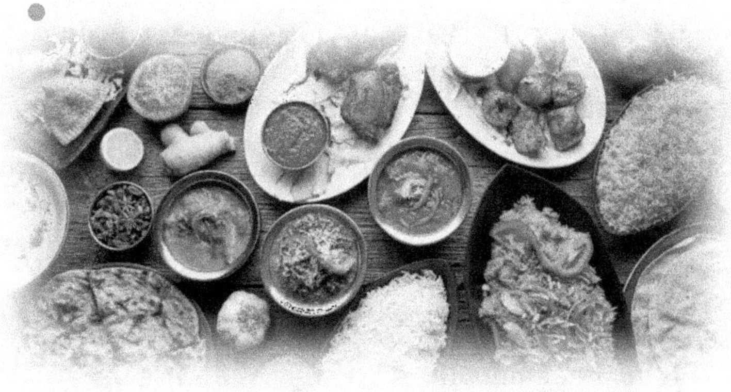

Conclusion

It is common knowledge that taking vitamin supplements on a regular basis has many positive effects on our bodies.

They not only maintain our bodies in good working order, but they also keep us healthy and prevent illness from striking readily.

Nevertheless, if we take them improperly, they may also have negative effects. Here are some safety precautions to follow when taking supplements.

Take Only as Directed

Prior to using vitamin supplements, we must read the directions on the packaging. This is the place where dosage and other information is stated.

If we don't, we might not be able to get the most out of the supplement or, worse, we might overdose.

Seek Your Doctor's Advice

It would be wise to see your doctor before taking any supplements. This is particularly true if you already use other medications.

If there is a chance that taking the supplement along with them could have negative consequences, your doctor can let you know. The same holds true if you have unique requirements for a specific vitamin.

Depending on the diagnosis, the physician can suggest taking it in larger amounts.

<u>Verify That It's Real</u>

Even if there are a lot of trustworthy supplements available, some are nonetheless fraudulent, ineffective, or both. They might do you more harm than good, so be cautious around them.

if you take vitamin supplements wrongly, they may be hazardous to you. Thus, do your research and confirm that the medication you are taking is safe.

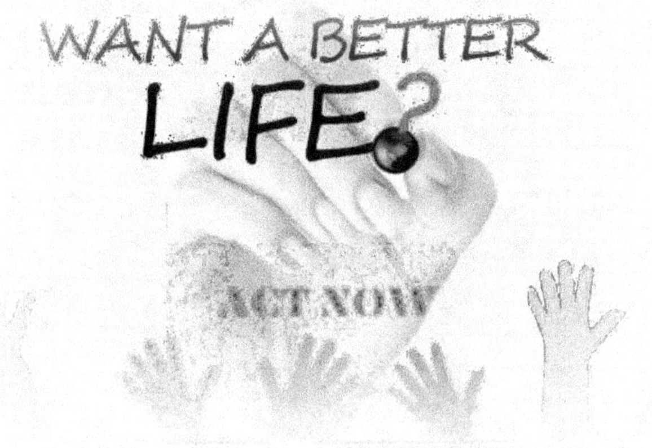

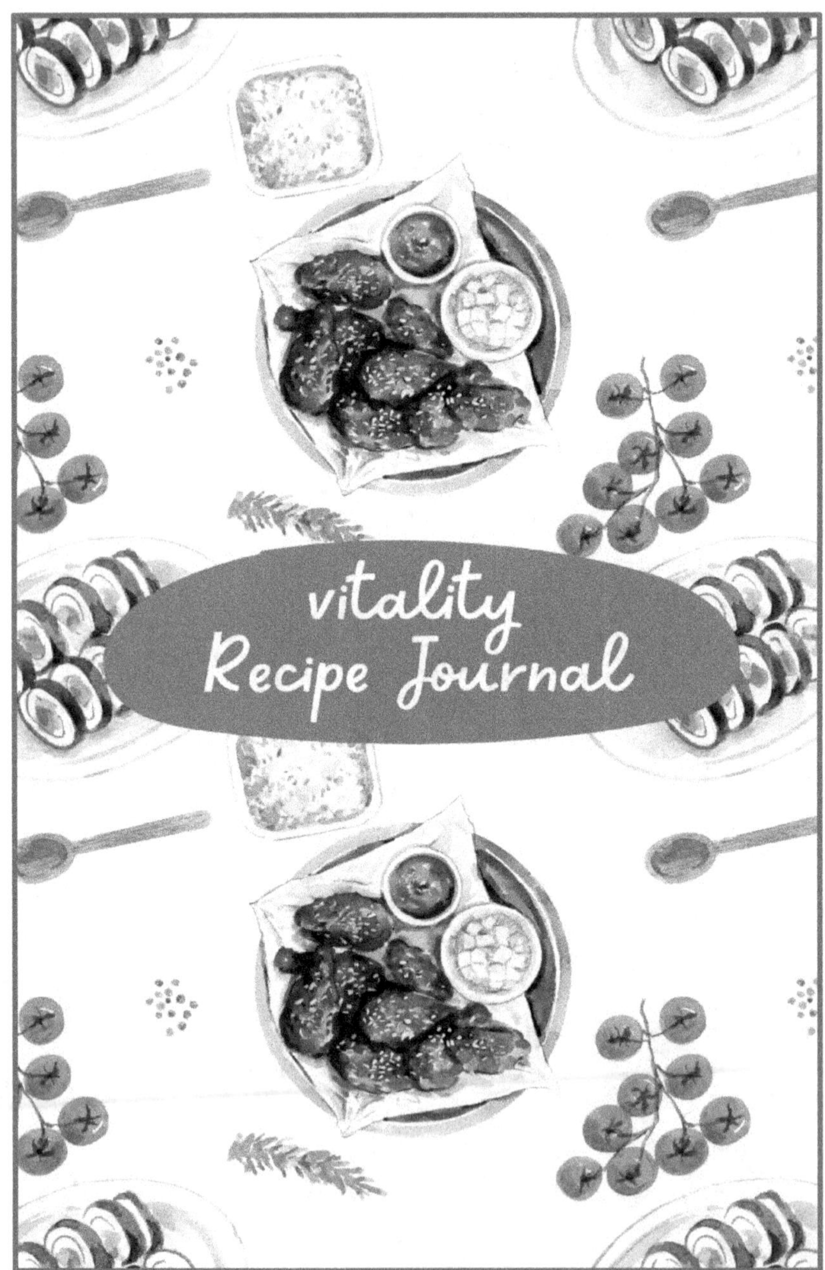
vitality
Recipe Journal

VITALITY LIFE-STYLE

WEEK:

Breakfast

Rate your day ○○○○○

Lunch

Rate your day ○○○○○

Dinner

Rate your day ○○○○○

Snacks

Rate your day ○○○○○

INGREDIENTS

NOTES:

VITALITY LIFE-STYLE

WEEK:

Breakfast

Rate your day ○○○○○

Lunch

Rate your day ○○○○○

Dinner

Rate your day ○○○○○

Snacks

Rate your day ○○○○○

INGREDIENTS

NOTES:

VITALITY LIFE-STYLE

WEEK:

Breakfast

Rate your day   ○ ○ ○ ○ ○

Lunch

Rate your day   ○ ○ ○ ○ ○

Dinner

Rate your day   ○ ○ ○ ○ ○

Snacks

Rate your day   ○ ○ ○ ○ ○

INGREDIENTS

NOTES:

VITALITY LIFE-STYLE

WEEK:

Breakfast

Rate your day ○○○○○

Lunch

Rate your day ○○○○○

Dinner

Rate your day ○○○○○

Snacks

Rate your day ○○○○○

INGREDIENTS

NOTES:

VITALITY LIFE-STYLE

WEEK:

Breakfast

Rate your day ○○○○○

INGREDIENTS

Lunch

Rate your day ○○○○○

Dinner

Rate your day ○○○○○

Snacks

Rate your day ○○○○○

VITALITY LIFE-STYLE

WEEK:

Breakfast

Rate your day ○○○○○

Lunch

Rate your day ○○○○○

Dinner

Rate your day ○○○○○

Snacks

Rate your day ○○○○○

INGREDIENTS

NOTES:

VITALITY LIFE-STYLE

WEEK:

Breakfast

Rate your day ○○○○○

Lunch

Rate your day ○○○○○

Dinner

Rate your day ○○○○○

Snacks

Rate your day ○○○○○

INGREDIENTS

NOTES:

VITALITY LIFE-STYLE

WEEK:

Breakfast

Rate your day   ○○○○○

Lunch

Rate your day   ○○○○○

Dinner

Rate your day   ○○○○○

Snacks

Rate your day   ○○○○○

INGREDIENTS

NOTES:

VITALITY LIFE-STYLE

WEEK:

Breakfast

Rate your day ○○○○○

Lunch

Rate your day ○○○○○

Dinner

Rate your day ○○○○○

Snacks

Rate your day ○○○○○

INGREDIENTS

NOTES:

VITALITY LIFE-STYLE

WEEK:

Breakfast

Rate your day ○○○○○

Lunch

Rate your day ○○○○○

Dinner

Rate your day ○○○○○

Snacks

Rate your day ○○○○○

INGREDIENTS

NOTES:

www.ingramcontent.com/pod-product-compliance
Lightning Source LLC
Chambersburg PA
CBHW050658250726
48662CB00002B/754